The Preschool  ory of P ess

Manual

Barbara Dodd and Sharon Crosbie
University of Newcastle upon Tyne, United Kingdom

Beth McIntosh, Tania Teitzel and Anne Ozanne
University of Queensland, Australia

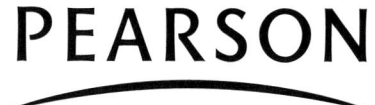

pipa

Published by Pearson Assessment, 80 Strand, London WC2R 0RL.
Copyright © 2000 Pearson Education, Inc. or its affiliate(s).
All rights reserved. No part of the publication may be reproduced or transmitted in any form or by any means, electronic or mechanical, including photocopy, recording or any information storage or retrieval system, without permission in writing from the publisher.
Printed in the United Kingdom.   ISBN 978 0 74911766 5

F G H 10 11 12

Contents

Acknowledgements	vii
List of subtests and equipment	ix
Chapter 1. Introduction	**1**
Purpose and uses of the PIPA	1
Test rationale	1
Phonological awareness	2
Development of phonological awareness	2
Preschool and Primary Inventory of Phonological Awareness	3
Test description	4
Subtest design	4
Syllable Segmentation	4
Rhyme Awareness	5
Alliteration Awareness	6
Phoneme Isolation	6
Phoneme Segmentation	7
Letter Knowledge	7
Chapter 2. Administration	**9**
General instructions	9
Test materials	9
Examiners	9
Testing procedures	9
Seating	10
Schedule of presentation	10
Calculating chronological age	10
Scoring	11
Basals and ceilings	11
Instructions for subtest administration and scoring	12
Syllable Segmentation	12
Rhyme Awareness	13
Alliteration Awareness	14
Phoneme Isolation	15
Phoneme Segmentation	16
Letter Knowledge	17
Chapter 3. Test interpretation	**19**
Calculating the standard scores and percentiles	19
Interpreting the scores	19

Contents

Chapter 4. Technical information ... 21
    Standardisation and normative sample ... 21
    Reliability ... 23
        Internal consistency ... 23
        Test-retest ... 23
        Inter-rater ... 24
    Validity ... 24
        Content validity ... 24
        Concurrent validity ... 25
        Criterion-related validity ... 25
        Construct validity ... 26

Chapter 5. Individual case studies ... 27
    Children with age appropriate phonological awareness skills ... 27
    Children at risk of literacy problems ... 29

References ... 33

Appendix A. Subtest standard scores (UK) ... 36
Appendix B. Subtest standard scores (Australia) ... 40
Appendix C. Confidence intervals +/- standard score points (UK) ... 44
Appendix D. Percentile ranks corresponding to standard scores ... 45

Figures
    Figure 2.1 Example of calculation of chronological age ... 10
    Figure 3.1 The normal curve and PIPA subtest standard scores and
        percentile ranks ... 20

Tables
    Table 1.1 Breakdown of skills by subtest ... 2
    Table 1.2 Age criteria for subtest assessment ... 4
    Table 1.3 Item analysis for Syllable Segmentation ... 5
    Table 1.4 Item analysis for Rhyme Awareness ... 5
    Table 1.5 Item analysis for Alliteration Awareness ... 6
    Table 1.6 Item analysis for Phoneme Isolation ... 6
    Table 1.7 Item analysis for Phoneme Segmentation ... 7
    Table 1.8 Item analysis for Letter Knowledge ... 7
    Table 3.1 Relationships between PIPA subtest standard scores,
        deviations from the mean and percentile ranks ... 20
    Table 4.1 Australian normative sample by age ... 21
    Table 4.2 Australian normative sample by gender ... 21
    Table 4.3 Australian normative sample by socio-economic status ... 21
    Table 4.4 United Kingdom normative sample by age ... 22

Table 4.5 United Kingdom normative sample by gender	22
Table 4.6 United Kingdom normative sample by socio-economic status	22
Table 4.7 United Kingdom normative sample by geographical area	22
Table 4.8 Internal consistency reliability coefficients for PIPA subtests	23
Table 4.9 Test-retest correlations for PIPA subtests	24
Table 4.10 PIPA test-retest t-values	24
Table 4.11 Correlations between PIPA and PAT scores on two subtests	25
Table 4.12 Correlations between the TERA and PIPA subtests	26
Table 4.13 Inter-correlations of the PIPA subtests	26

Appendix A
Subtest standard scores (UK) 3:0-3:5	36
Subtest standard scores (UK) 3:6-3:11	36
Subtest standard scores (UK) 4:0-4:5	37
Subtest standard scores (UK) 4:6-4:11	37
Subtest standard scores (UK) 5:0-5:5	38
Subtest standard scores (UK) 5:6-5:11	38
Subtest standard scores (UK) 6:0-6:5	39
Subtest standard scores (UK) 6:6-6:11	39

Appendix B
Subtest standard scores (Australia) 3:0-3:5	40
Subtest standard scores (Australia) 3:6-3:11	40
Subtest standard scores (Australia) 4:0-4:5	41
Subtest standard scores (Australia) 4:6-4:11	41
Subtest standard scores (Australia) 5:0-5:5	42
Subtest standard scores (Australia) 5:6-3:11	42
Subtest standard scores (Australia) 6:0-6:5	43
Subtest standard scores (Australia) 6:6-6:11	43

Appendix C
Confidence intervals +/- standard score points (UK)	44

Appendix D
Percentile ranks corresponding to standard scores	45

Acknowledgements

We would like to thank:

The many children, parents and schools who agreed to participate in the norming of the Preschool and Primary Inventory of Phonological Awareness (PIPA).

The undergraduate and postgraduate students of University of Newcastle upon Tyne who contributed to the development of the PIPA, especially Ruth Houlton and Margaret Coates who assisted with validity and reliability studies.

Professor David Howard for assistance with statistical analysis of the data.

The development of the PIPA was resourced by the National Health and Medical Research Council of Australia.

List of subtests and equipment

Subtests involved

	Subtest	Equipment needed
Subtest 1	Syllable Segmentation	Stimulus Booklet
Subtest 2	Rhyme Awareness	Stimulus Booklet
Subtest 3	Alliteration Awareness	Stimulus Booklet
Subtest 4	Phoneme Isolation	Stimulus Booklet
Subtest 5	Phoneme Segmentation	Stimulus Booklet, counters
Subtest 6	Letter Knowledge	Stimulus Booklet

Equipment enclosed

25 Record Forms
Stimulus Booklet

Necessary equipment not included

5 counters
Pen
Tape recorder and blank tape (optional)

Chapter 1
Introduction

Purpose and uses of the PIPA

The Preschool and Primary Inventory of Phonological Awareness (PIPA) was designed to identify children who have poor phonological awareness. The link between phonological awareness in the preschool years and the later successful development of literacy skills necessitates a reliable and quick assessment tool for preliterate children. The PIPA can also be used as a means of measuring change in phonological awareness. The 6 sound awareness skills evaluated by the PIPA are: syllable segmentation, rhyme awareness, alliteration awareness, phoneme (sound) isolation, phoneme segmentation and letter knowledge. All of the subtests were constructed to meet the following criteria:

- to assess areas of sound knowledge in 3 to 7 year old children;

- to be a 'pure' test of the relevant skills being evaluated;

- to be able to be administered separately to explore specific sound awareness skills as required;

- to be easy to administer and allow for flexibility of testing; and,

- the picture stimuli must be colourful and interesting.

Test rationale

Preliterate measures of phonological awareness predict early reading and spelling skills more accurately than any other single variable including intelligence scores, age and socio-economic status (Bryant, MacLean, Bradley, & Crossland, 1990). Early identification of children with poor phonological awareness would allow appropriate intervention to be offered that might prevent reading and spelling failure and the negative consequences commonly associated with literacy difficulties. There is a need, then, to develop standardised assessments of phonological awareness for preliterate children.

Chapter 1

Phonological awareness

Phonological awareness refers to knowledge about the sound structure of the language and the skill to manipulate sound units. Read (1971) demonstrated that preschool children have an implicit knowledge of the internal structure of words. However, the acquisition of alphabetic literacy requires children's implicit knowledge of the phonological structure of words to be made explicit (McCormick, 1995). Phonological awareness is not a unitary skill (Hoien, Lundberg, Stanovich, & Bjaalid, 1995). Words can be broken down into smaller units in at least three ways:

- *Syllabic:* The awareness of syllables in words. (e.g. door: /dx/; daughter: /dx - tx/; democracy: /dx - mo - krx - si/)

- *Intra-syllabic:* The awareness of onset and rime. The onset consists of the initial consonant or consonant cluster, and the rime the vowel and any proceeding consonants. (e.g. door: /d - x/; dog: /d - og/; drum: /dr - xm/)

- *Phonemic:* The awareness of individual sounds in words. (e.g. door: /d - x; dog: /d - o - g/; daughter: /d -x - t - x/)

Awareness of these three levels of phonological units can be measured by subtests that investigate the ability to detect, segment or manipulate the units at the specified level. Different subtests involve different cognitive skills, and there is a developmental progression according to the complexity of the subtest.

Table 1.1 Breakdown of skills by subtest

Operation	Phonological Awareness Level		
	Syllable	Onset-rime	Phoneme
Detect		Rhyme Awareness	Alliteration Awareness
Isolate	Syllable Segmentation	Phoneme Isolation	Phoneme Segmentation
Manipulate			
Conversion			Letter Knowledge

Development of phonological awareness

Phonological awareness develops along a continuum: awareness of larger units is developed prior to awareness of smaller units (Caravolas & Bruck, 1993). Awareness of the syllabic unit is attained early. Perhaps it is the easiest to detect because each syllable unit is a salient peak of acoustic energy (Liberman, Shankweiler, Fischer, & Carter, 1974). Intra-syllabic awareness skills are the next to emerge. A strong relationship has been established between the knowledge of nursery rhymes and the development of awareness of onsets and rimes (Maclean, Bryant, & Bradley, 1987). This finding suggests that the awareness of intra-syllabic units is not a natural cognitive achievement but is developed through linguistic experience.

Phonemic awareness is strongly related to the ability to read an alphabet. Most children are unable to perform phonemic awareness tasks before exposure to writing, and consequently this level of awareness is not usually present in preschool children. Treiman and Baron (1981) claimed that, 'To most adults, it is obvious that spoken words consist of smaller units. To young children, however, these insights do not come easily. [Preliterate] children typically have trouble on tasks that demand a sensitivity to the number of segments in a spoken word.' (p.159). To acquire alphabetic literacy the child must begin to realise that letters represent individual speech sounds, and in turn, strings of letters represent the strings of sounds that make up a word (Goswami & Bryant, 1990).

Preschool and Primary Inventory of Phonological Awareness

The battery of subtests used in the PIPA assess the three principle components of phonological awareness identified by Hoien *et al.* (1995) of syllable, onset-rime and phoneme awareness. Yopp (1988) found that rhyme detection, alliteration detection, phoneme isolation and phoneme segmentation each demonstrated high construct validity. Phoneme isolation and segmentation have the best predictive validity for later reading (Yopp, 1988; Liberman & Shankweiler, 1985). Letter recognition is a prerequisite for alphabetic literacy.

Increasing interest in the phonological awareness abilities of preliterate children argues the need for a range of formal, standardised assessments for research and clinical practice. For example, while research has established that awareness of the segments in the acoustic speech stream predicts alphabetic literacy, the nature of that relationship has yet to be completely understood (Passenger, Stuart & Terrell, 2000). Most published investigations into phonological awareness skills have used different experimental tasks and as a result a vast array of unstandardised tests has accumulated (McBride-Chang, 1995). Standardised assessment tests are useful research tools, allowing comparison between children with typical and atypical learning abilities and from differing environments.

Training phonological awareness has recently been introduced as an intervention approach for children with both spoken and written disabilities (Dodd & Gillon, 1997). Children as young as three years can be involved in programmes that focus on aspects of phonological awareness. However, there is little evidence concerning the age at which phonological awareness skills typically emerge. While there is a consensus concerning the order of emergence, normative data on the age of emergence, and course of development of specific phonological skills in the preschool years, is not well established. Standardised tests can provide important benchmarks for diagnosis of phonological awareness deficits.

Test description

The PIPA consists of six subtests: five assess different aspects of phonological (sound) awareness and one test of grapheme-phoneme knowledge (the letter sounds). Each subtest takes 4–5 minutes to administer. The test can be completed in 25-30 minutes. Normative data is provided for each subtest so it is possible to administer the complete test or individual subtests.

Table 1.2. Age criteria for subtest assessment

Below 4 years of age	From 4 years of age
Rhyme Awareness	Rhyme Awareness
Syllable Segmentation	Syllable Segmentation
Alliteration Awareness	Alliteration Awareness
	Phoneme Isolation
	Phoneme Segmentation
	Letter Knowledge

Subtest Design

Each PIPA subtest is designed to assess different aspects of phonological awareness development. The following section describes the design and test format for each subtest.

Syllable Segmentation

The Syllable Segmentation subtest assesses the child's ability to process words at a sub-lexical level. It is the first phonological awareness skill to emerge (Liberman, Shankweiler, Fischer, & Carter, 1974). The ability to segment syllables is important for analysing words for spelling and reading (Rack, Snowling & Olsen, 1992).

There are 4 practice items and 12 test items spoken by the examiner. The test items have been chosen so that they are unlikely to be in the child's vocabulary (e.g., periodical). The string cannot be segmented on the basis of a phonological representation accessed from the lexicon but must be stored and analysed in phonological working memory (Gathercole & Baddeley, 1993).

Item analysis is by syllable length (two to five syllables included).

Table 1.3. Item analysis for Syllable Segmentation

No. of syllables	Items			
2	1		6	8
3	2		5	12
4	3		7	9
5	4		10	11

Rhyme Awareness

Rhyme awareness reflects children's ability to judge phonological similarity of spoken words. Sensitivity to rhyme and the ability to identify rimes have been shown to affect a child's ability to acquire literacy skills. It is particularly important for spelling as it underlies the ability to use analogy to spell unfamiliar words (Goswami & Bryant, 1990). The emergence of the ability to detect rhyme signals that children are able to analyse words at an intrasyllabic level.

This subtest requires the child to choose the word that does not rhyme from a set of four words (adapted from Bradley & Bryant, 1983). The test items are spoken by the examiner and supported by picture stimuli to reduce memory load. There are 2 practice items and 12 test items. The items chosen were simple, highly imageable, one syllable words. Item analysis for Rhyme Awareness is by the position of the non-rhyming word to identify any strategies a child may use to complete the subtest (e.g., child always selects last picture).

Table 1.4. Item analysis for Rhyme Awareness

Position	Items			
First	4		6*	10
Second	8		9	11*
Third	3		7	12*
Last	1*		2	5

* Item has alliterative distracters

Chapter 1

Alliteration Awareness

Alliteration awareness reflects children's ability to segment at an intra-syllabic level and compare similarity of onsets. It predicts later single word reading (Passenger, Stuart & Terell, 2000). An awareness of onsets precedes the ability to name initial sounds in words (Burt, Holm & Dodd, 1999).

This subtest requires the child to choose the word that does not start with the same sound from a set of four words. The test items are spoken by the examiner and supported by picture stimuli. There are 2 practice items and 12 test items ranging from one to three syllables. Item analysis is by the position of the 'odd one out' to identify any strategies a child may use to complete the subtest.

Table 1.5. Item analysis for Alliteration Awareness

Position	Items			
First	6	8	9	
Second	2	7	12	
Third	3	5	10	
Last	1	4	11	

Phoneme Isolation

Phoneme isolation reflects children's ability to recognise onsets, segment them from the rime and pronounce an isolated sound. The ability to isolate sounds was shown by Yopp (1988) to be one of the best predictors for the ability to sound and blend non-words.

The stimuli are spoken by the examiner and supported by picture stimuli. Children are asked to respond with the first sound. There is one demonstration, two practice items and 12 test items. The item analysis for Phoneme Isolation distinguishes between single graphemes, digraphs and clusters.

Table 1.6. Item analysis for Phoneme Isolation

Category	Items				
Single consonant sound/ grapheme	1	2	6	9	10
Single consonant sound/ digraph	8	11			
Vowel	4	12			
Part of a cluster	3	5	7		

Phoneme Segmentation

Phoneme segmentation is a reliable predictor of early reading and spelling ability (Muter, Hulme, Snowling & Taylor, 1998). Segmenting phonemes is more difficult than segmenting onset-rimes (Yopp, 1988). It is an essential skill for plausibly spelling unfamiliar words.

This subtest requires the child to segment a spoken word into individual phonemes. There are 2 demonstration items, 4 practice items and 12 test items. Item analysis is by number of phonemes.

Table 1.7. Item analysis for Phoneme Segmentation

Phonemes	One:One	One:Many
2		1 5 8
3		3 9 12
4	10 11	6
5	2	4 7

Letter Knowledge

The ability to decode letters to their corresponding phoneme shows children's grasp of the alphabetic nature of the written language (Johnston & Watson, 1997). Segmenting phonemes without linking it to letter knowledge would not allow an individual to progress beyond logographic literacy. Teaching grapheme-phoneme correspondences has been shown to accelerate the acquisition of literacy (Stuart, 1999).

This subtest requires the child to say a sound when presented with a letter. There are 2 practice items and 32 test items. Test items include single grapheme-phoneme correspondence, digraphs, clusters and vowels (monothongs and dipthongs).

Table 1.8. Item analysis for Letter Knowledge

Item category	Items				
Single grapheme	1	4	6	10	13
	15	16	17	18	19
	20	21	23	24	26
	29	30	31	32	
Digraph	2	5	8		
Cluster	11	22	25	27	28
Vowel monothong	3	7	9	12	14

Chapter 2
Administration

General Instructions

Test materials

The PIPA materials required are:

- *Manual.* This manual contains a description of the theory on which the test is based, test design and development information, procedures for administering, scoring and interpreting the test, the normative data, and appendices.

- *Stimulus Booklet.* This booklet contains the visual stimuli needed to administer the assessment.

- *Record Form.*

- 5 Counters (to be supplied by examiner).

Examiners

The PIPA was designed for speech and language therapists, teachers and professionals assessing children's early literacy skills. Examiners who give and interpret the test should have experience in standardised test administration, scoring, interpretation and assessing children.

Testing procedures

To ensure a reliable administration of the PIPA the examiner should:

- be familiar with the *Manual* and *Stimulus Booklet*;

- administer the test individually in a quiet, well lit room;

- establish rapport with the child prior to the assessment;

- provide appropriate non-specific feedback to the child throughout testing. This includes making general comments such as 'well done', 'only a few more to go' and 'aren't you clever to do all this work'. Comments that focus on the child's test performance should be avoided, e.g., 'that's right' or 'that's not right';

- record responses accurately and audio record if necessary;
- adhere to the guidelines for administration; and,
- have the *Stimulus Booklet, Record Form,* pencil, audio recorder and audio cassette available when testing.

The examiner may point to the individual picture stimuli while saying the item name in all trial and test items.

Seating

Sit next to the child so that the stimulus material is clearly visible to both of you. If you are right handed sit on the child's right side. If you are left handed sit on the child's left side so that you can record responses and turn the pages of the *Stimulus Booklet*.

Schedule of presentation

The subtests in the PIPA may be administered in any order. Some subtest formats are similar and so these subtests should not be administered in succession. These subtests are:

- Rhyme Awareness and Alliteration Awareness
- Phoneme Segmentation and Syllable Segmentation

Calculating chronological age

Before commencing the test, complete the child's information details on the *Record Form* and calculate the child's chronological age. To calculate a child's chronological age subtract the child's birth date from the test date. Remember to always borrow 30 days from the month and 12 months from the year when completing calculations. For example:

Figure 2.1. Example of calculatiion of chronological age.

	Year	Month	Day
Test date	2000	~~3~~ 2	~~19~~ 49
Birth date	1995	1	23
Chronological age	5	1	26

Scoring

Details for scoring each subtest are found on the *Record Form*. To compute the raw scores for the subtest add the scores of the individual items administered.

Basals and ceilings

The examiner does not need to be concerned with establishing basals as all subtests begin with the first item. Ceilings are established when the discontinuation criteria for each subtest are met. These are listed on the *Record Form*. If the test was discontinued, the last item scoring greater than 0 is considered the ceiling.

Chapter 2

Instructions for subtest administration and scoring

Syllable Segmentation

Picture stimuli	Record Form	Repetitions	Age	Discontinue rule
Stimulus Booklet	Page 2	One allowed	All ages	Administer all items

Instructions

Say

> When we say words we can say them in drumbeats (demonstrate by tapping the appropriate number of drums or clapping the syllables). We can say ELEPHANT like this: EL...E...PHANT. Now you do it. (Provide appropriate feedback.)
>
> Now you tap out,   puppy   rhinoceros   vestibule   originator

Continue on to the test items but do not provide feedback.

Scoring

Record the child's responses. Score according to the child's oral segmentation NOT the drums they point to or number of claps they make. Score 1 if all of the syllables are segmented, 0 for an incorrect response and NR for no response.

Administration

Rhyme Awareness

Picture stimuli	Record Form	Repetitions	Age	Discontinue rule
Stimulus Booklet	Page 3	One allowed	All ages	Administer all items

Instructions

Say

> Do you know Humpty Dumpty? Humpty Dumpty sat on a WALL, Humpty Dumpty had a great FALL. Listen WALL – FALL sound the same. They rhyme. Let's find another one that sounds the same as WALL and FALL. WALL – FALL – BALL. BALL sounds the same. It rhymes. WALL – FALL – BALL – CAT. CAT doesn't sound like WALL – FALL – BALL. It doesn't belong.
>
> We're going to play a game with some more words that sound the same. Listen to the words. Show me the picture that doesn't belong.
>
> * WALL – FALL – BALL – CAT. Administer as above. Provide feedback.
>
> * FEET – SHEET – SEAT – KEY. Which one doesn't belong? Provide feedback.

Continue on to the test items but do not provide feedback.

Scoring

Score 1 for each correct response, 0 for an incorrect response and NR for no response.

Chapter 2

Alliteration Awareness

Picture stimuli	Record Form	Repetitions	Age	Discontinue rule
Stimulus Booklet	Page 4	One allowed	All ages	Administer all items

Instructions

Say

Your name, (say child's name) starts with a (say initial sound of name). I know other words that start with a (initial sound), (say two words that share same initial sound). I'm going to say all the words again but this time I'm going to say another word that starts with a different sound. Say all of the previously mentioned words and a word with different onset.

Say

(Word with different onset) starts with a (sound). It doesn't belong.

Now let's look at the pictures in the book. Three of the words start with the same sound. One doesn't. See if you can work out which one doesn't belong.

LEAF – LIGHT – LAKE – CAT. Which one doesn't belong? Provide feedback.

HEAD – HOUSE – BIRD – HAT. Which one doesn't belong? Provide feedback.

Continue on to the test items but do not provide feedback.

Scoring

Score 1 for each correct response, 0 for an incorrect response and NR for no response.

Administration

Phoneme Isolation

Picture stimuli	Record Form	Repetitions	Age	Discontinue rule
Stimulus Booklet	Page 4	One allowed	4 years and above	4 consecutive errors

Instructions

Say

> The first sound of your name is ... (expect child to say initial sound and provide praise. Say initial sound if child does not respond). Here is a picture of a DOG. The first sound of DOG is /d/. Let's try some others.
>
> * Tell me the first sound of APPLE. Provide appropriate feedback.
>
> * Tell me the first sound of BALL. Provide appropriate feedback.

Continue on to the test items but do not provide feedback.

Scoring

Record the child's responses. Score 1 for each correct response (initial sound with or without a schwa vowel), 0 for an incorrect response and NR for no response.

Phoneme Segmentation

Materials	Record Form	Repetitions	Age	Discontinue rule
Stimulus Booklet Counters	Page 6	One allowed	4 years and above	4 consecutive errors

Instructions

Say

Here's a BEAR. We can say BEAR like this with counters B...EAR. (Separate each sound and place appropriate number of counters on page). Now you show me. Provide appropriate feedback. Let's try another one - PIG. I'm going to say PIG with counters, P...I...G. This time you're going to do it without the pictures.

Show me,   UP (2)   BOAT (3)   MUM (3)   PUPPY (4)

Continue on to the test items but do not provide feedback.

Scoring

Record the child's responses. The child is required to clearly separate each sound as scoring is dependent on oral segmentation NOT the number of counters they use. Score 1 for each correct response (all phonemes segmented), 0 for an incorrect response and NR for no response.

Letter Knowledge

Picture stimuli	Record Form	Repetitions	Age	Discontinue rule
Stimulus Booklet	Page 7	One allowed	4 years and above	See below

Instructions

Say

Do you know what sound this letter makes? Examiner points to 's'. It says /s/. Say sound. What about this one? Examiner points to 'm'. Provide feedback.

If the child says the letter name, say That's its name but what sound does it make?

We're going to look at some more letters. You say what sound they make.

Continue on to the test items but do not provide feedback.

Point to each letter in turn moving from left to right along each line. Start at the top line and move down the page. Children who belong in the younger age groups may be shown the letters one line at a time.

If the child does not say a sound within approximately 5 seconds move to the next item. If the child has not been able to say the sound of 10 consecutive items then say Look at this page. Are there any ones that you know? Repeat for second page if required.

Scoring

Score 1 for each correct response, 0 for an incorrect response and NR for no response.

Chapter 3
Test interpretation

Calculating the standard scores and percentiles

1. After completing each subtest transfer the child's raw subtest scores to the summary sheet on page 1 of the *Record Form*.

2. Convert the raw score into a normalised standard score using Appendix A (UK children) OR Appendix B (Australian children). Locate the table for the child's chronological age. The raw scores for each subtest are presented in columns. Search for the child's raw subtest score in the body of the table. The corresponding standard score is listed in the left hand column.

3. Look up the corresponding percentile scores presented in Appendix D.

4. Optional: Establish confidence intervals from Appendix C (UK children only). Locate the age group in column 1 and choose the preferred level of confidence (68% or 95%). For each subtest in the age group locate the interval expressed in +/- standard score points. Add this number to the standard score, then subtract this same number from the standard score. These two scores represent the upper and lower limits for a child. For example: A child aged 4 years:8 months obtains a standard score of 9 on Syllable Segmentation. Points specified at the 68% confidence levels are 1.2. The confidence interval is therefore 7.8 (9 - 1.2) to 10.2 (9 + 1.2).

Interpreting the scores

A standard score of 10 is the mean and there is a standard deviation (SD) of 3. Approximately two-thirds of all children earn subtest standard scores between 7 and 13, i.e., within 1SD of the mean. This range is considered to denote normal phonological awareness skills.

Each standard score can also be expressed as a percentile rank. See Appendix D for conversion table from standard scores to percentile ranks.

A standard score of 10 equates to a percentile score of 50. The 50th percentile is the score below which 50% of the scores in the distribution of the standardisation sample fall. Figure 3.1 shows the relationship between PIPA subtest standard scores and a normal distribution of scores. Table 3.1 shows the

Chapter 3

relationship between PIPA subtest standard scores, deviations from the mean and percentile ranks.

Confidence intervals are based on the psychometric standard error of measurement (SEM). The scores obtained allow for the measurement error inherent in all tests and reflects the likelihood (at either a 68% or 95% level of confidence) that the child's true score falls within this range. A range of scores rather than a single value is useful when making important placement decisions based on the test results.

Subtest raw scores, standard scores and percentile ranks can be transferred to the Score Summary section on page 1 of the *Record Form*. Completion of the Profile graph on page 1 of the *Record Form* will provide a visual summary of the child's overall performance, and indicate strengths and weaknesses in subtest performance.

Table 3.1. Relationship between PIPA subtest standard scores, deviations from the mean and percentile ranks

Subtest standard score	Standard deviations from the mean	Percentile Rank
19	+3	99
16	+2	98
13	+1	84
10	0 (mean)	50
7	-1	16
4	-2	2
1	-3	1

Figure 3.1. The normal curve and PIPA subtest standard scores and percentile ranks

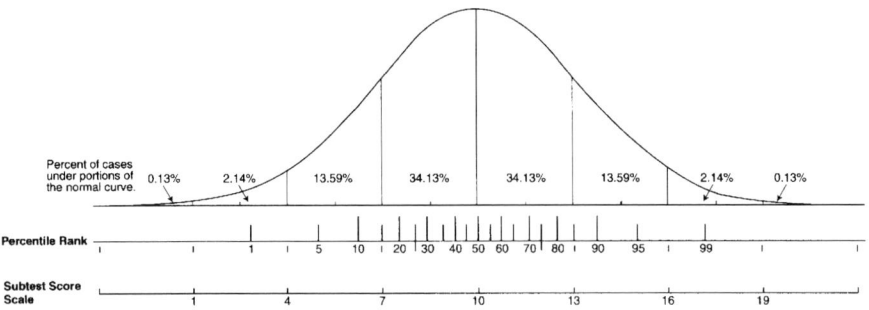

Copyright © 1990 by The Psychological Corporation. Adapted with permission. All rights reserved

Chapter 4

Technical information

Standardisation and normative sample

A goal in the development of the PIPA was to allow norm-referenced comparisons of a child's performance to the performance of normally achieving children of the same age. The initial PIPA standardisation study was conducted in Brisbane, Australia in 1995 and 1996. It included 583 children between the ages of 3 years and 6 years: 11 months. Testing was carried out by two paediatric speech and language therapists. Demographic characteristics of the sample are shown in tables 4.1, 4.2 and 4.3.

Table 4.1. Australian normative sample by age

Age group (years:months)	n	Mean age (years:months)	SD
3:0-3:5	71	3:3.0	1.7
3:6-3:11	79	3:8.9	1.9
4:0-4:5	76	4:2.6	1.8
4:6-4:11	78	4:9.0	1.7
5:0-5:5	75	5:2.4	1.8
5:6-5:11	64	5:9.2	1.6
6:0-6:5	66	6:3.0	1.6
6:6-6:11	74	6:8.6	1.8

Table 4.2. Australian normative sample by gender

Gender	n	% of sample
Male	276	47.3
Female	307	52.7

Table 4.3. Australian normative sample by socio-economic status (SES)

SES	n	% of sample
Low	190	32.6
Mid	200	34.3
High	193	33.1

During 1999 the PIPA, with the addition of the subtest *Letter Knowledge*, was given to 595 children between the ages of 3:0 and 6:11 years in the United Kingdom. Testing was carried out by undergraduate and postgraduate students at the University of Newcastle after training. Most testing was carried out during the summer vacation near the students' home town. Examiners were required to sample across the age range of the sample to balance any bias in test procedure. Only native English speaking children not currently attending speech therapy were included in the large normative sample. Demographic characteristics of the sample are shown in tables 4.4, 4.5, 4.6 and 4.7.

Table 4.4. United Kingdom normative sample by age

Age group (years:months)	n	Mean age (years:months)	SD
3:0–3:5	27	3:2.5	1.6
3:6–3:11	54	3:8.8	1.7
4:0–4:5	55	4:2.2	1.8
4:6–4:11	107	4:9.2	1.6
5:0–5:5	94	5:2.5	1.6
5:6–5:11	97	5:8.5	1.6
6:0–6:5	78	6:2.7	1.7
6:6–6:11	83	6:10.4	1.8

Table 4.5. United Kingdom normative sample by gender

Gender	n	% of sample
Male	277	47.0
Female	317	53.0

Table 4.6. United Kingdom normative sample by socio-economic status (SES)

SES	n	% of sample
Low	381	64.0
Mid	210	36.0

Table 4.7. United Kingdom normative sample by geographical area

	n	% of sample
North	223	37.5
Midlands	143	24.0
South	114	19.2
West	115	19.3
Total	595	100.0

Reliability

The precision and consistency with which the PIPA measures the performance of an individual must be evident when a score is used to make decisions about the need for intervention. The following methods were used to evaluate the reliability of the PIPA:

- Internal consistency
- Test-retest reliability
- Inter-rater reliability

Internal consistency

Internal consistency reliability coefficients describe the precision of scores on a test. The use of internal consistency as a measure of reliability implies that the items within a test are homogenous. PIPA reliability coefficients for the UK sample were obtained using Cronbach's coefficient alpha. Internal consistency reliability coefficients are reported by subtest in Table 4.8. Alpha scores above 0.7 are considered acceptable.

Table 4.8. Internal consistency reliability coefficients for PIPA subtests

Subtest	Alpha
Syllable Segmentation	0.8393
Rhyme Awareness	0.8326
Alliteration Awareness	0.8420
Phoneme Isolation	0.9157
Phoneme Segmentation	0.7046*
Letter Knowledge	0.9756

* *The comparatively lower alpha reflects better performance on 2–3 phoneme items.*

Test-retest

The stability of PIPA scores was also assessed over time. The sample consisted of 42 children ranging from age 3 to 7 years with a mean age of 5:0 years. The between test interval was two weeks. Both tests were administered by the same examiner. The correlations obtained between the scores at test one and test two are given for the subtests in Table 4.9.

Chapter 4

Table 4.9. Test-retest correlations for PIPA subtests

Subtest	Pearson correlation
Syllable Segmentation	0.691
Rhyme Awareness	0.870
Alliteration Awareness	0.803
Phoneme Isolation	0.949
Phoneme Segmentation	0.326
Letter Knowledge	0.980

The test-retest reliability coefficients are acceptable indicating consistent performance on subtests over a period of time. The low, but significant correlation for phoneme segmentation suggests this subtest is less reliable than the other subtests.

Inter-rater

Most of the PIPA subtests are scored objectively. Nevertheless to ensure that two independent raters would score the child's performance in the same manner a small group of six children were videoed. A second speech and language pathologist rescored the test. Table 4.10 shows the results of independent t-tests of the scores recorded by the two examiners. There were no significant differences between the scorers.

Table 4.10. PIPA test-retest t-values

Subtest	t value	Significance (2-tailed)
Syllable Segmentation	-1.150	0.277
Rhyme Awareness	0.000	1.000
Alliteration Awareness	-0.143	0.889
Phoneme Isolation	-1.581	0.145
Phoneme Segmentation	-0.632	0.341
Letter Knowledge	0.099	0.923

Validity

Validity is the extent a test measures what it claims to measure. Research conducted with the PIPA provides evidence of content, concurrent, predictive and construct validity.

Content validity

Content validity evaluates whether the subtests in the PIPA are recognised measures of phonological awareness. Earlier in this manual the design of each PIPA subtest was described, including an analysis of specific subtest content. The phonological awareness skills assessed by the PIPA are well documented in the literature addressing phonological awareness. The subtests are based on research tests that have been shown to effectively identify phonological awareness deficits.

Concurrent validity

Concurrent validity refers to the correlation of the assessment with other tests known to be valid measures of the area. The concurrent validity of the PIPA was obtained by comparing scores obtained on another measure of phonological awareness; the Phonological Abilities Test (PAT) (Muter, Hulme & Snowling, 1997). Correlations compared the two subtests that are common to both tests; rhyme detection and letter knowledge. Table 4.11 shows that the scores from the PIPA and the PAT are significantly correlated, providing evidence that the PIPA has concurrent validity.

Table 4.11. Correlations between PIPA and PAT scores on two subtests

PIPA	PAT	
	Rhyme detection	Letter knowledge
Rhyme detection	0.631*	0.612*
Letter knowledge	0.590*	0.916*

* Correlation is significant at the 0.01 level (2 tailed)

Criterion-related validity

Criterion-related validity assesses the test's value as a predictor of performance in a relevant area. As the PIPA was designed to assist in the identification of children who have poor phonological awareness as it pertains to literacy, a measure of early reading development was judged to be the most appropriate criterion reference. Predictive validity refers to this aspect of criterion-related validity.

Criterion-related validity was evaluated by comparing speech disordered children's performance on the PIPA and the Test of Early Reading Ability (TERA) (Reid, Hresko & Hammill, 1989).

Thirty 4:0 to 6:4 year old children, referred to the University Speech and Language Therapy clinic in Brisbane, were evaluated on a standardised reading measure and the PIPA correlations between the TERA and five of the PIPA subtests are shown in Table 4.12.

Chapter 4

Table 4.12. Correlations between the TERA and PIPA subtests

	TERA correlations
Syllable Segmentation	0.440*
Rhyme Awareness	0.473**
Alliteration Awareness	0.499**
Phoneme Isolation	0.389*
Phoneme Segmentation	0.457*

*Correlation is significant at the 0.01 level (2 tailed).
**Correlation is significant at the 0.001 level (2 tailed).

Construct Validity

Construct validity refers to whether the subtests included in the assessment evaluate the named ability, for the PIPA, phonological awareness. One way of evaluating construct validity is by examining the intercorrelations among subtests. Table 4.13 presents the inter-correlations between subtests for the sample as a whole.

Table 4.13 Inter-correlations of the PIPA subtests

	SSeg	RA	AA	PI	PS	LK
Syllable Segmentation (SSeg)		0.416	0.414	0.462	0.327	0.485
Rhyme Awareness (RA)			0.703	0.604	0.539	0.672
Alliteration Awareness (AA)				0.645	0.588	0.728
Phoneme Isolation (PI)					0.556	0.788
Phoneme Segmentation (PS)						0.628
Letter Knowledge (LK)						

All correlations were significant at the 0.01 level (2-tailed). Letter knowledge was highly correlated with alliteration awareness, phoneme isolation and segmentation. There was a weaker correlation between syllable and phoneme segmentation. An interesting pattern in the UK normative data between 5:6 and 6 years indicates that children are less aware of syllables when they are exposed and explicitly learning about letters and sounds. This is reflected in a decrease in their ability to segment at a syllabic level and an increase in their intra-syllabic awareness.

Chapter 5
Individual case studies

Case studies of five typically developing children are presented. In addition three case studies are presented profiling the phonological awareness skills of two children with speech disorder and a child with literacy difficulties.

Children with age appropriate phonological awareness skills

Ella (aged 3 years: 10 months)

Ella had an age equivalent score on the Visual Motor Integration Test (Beery, 1989) of 4 years: 3 months. She lives in Essex in a middle SES area. No previous history of speech and language difficulties were reported.

Ella's scores on the PIPA subtests were:

Subtest	Raw score	Standard Score	Percentile
Syllable Segmentation	6/12	11	63
Rhyme Awareness	5/12	10	50
Alliteration Awareness	2/12	8	25

Ella scored age appropriately on all of the PIPA subtests.

Connor (aged 4 years: 2 months)

Connor had an age equivalent score on the Visual Motor Integration Test (Beery, 1989) of 4 years: 10 months. He lives in rural Yorkshire and no previous history of speech and language difficulties were reported.

Connor's scores on the PIPA subtests were:

Subtest	Raw score	Standard Score	Percentile
Syllable Segmentation	3/12	8	25
Rhyme Awareness	9/12	14	91
Alliteration Awareness	5/12	11	63
Phoneme Isolation	7/12	12	75
Phoneme Segmentation	0/12	8	25
Letter Knowledge	6/32	9	37

Connor performed at age appropriate levels on all of the PIPA subtests.

Chapter 5

Alex (aged 5 years: 1 month)

Alex had an age equivalent score on the Visual Motor Integration Test (Beery, 1989) of 4 years: 10 months. He lives in Scunthorpe in an area with a low SES. No previous history of speech and language difficulties were reported.

Alex's scores on the PIPA subtests were:

Subtest	Raw score	Standard Score	Percentile
Syllable Segmentation	11/12	13	84
Rhyme Awareness	9/12	12	75
Alliteration Awareness	12/12	14	91
Phoneme Isolation	10/12	11	63
Phoneme Segmentation	4/12	11	63
Letter Knowledge	24/32	11	63

Alex scored at the upper limits of the normal range on all of the PIPA subtests.

Emily (aged 5 years: 5 months)

Emily had an age equivalent score on the Visual Motor Integration Test (Beery, 1989) of 7 years: 8 months. She lives in a low SES area of Middlesbrough. No previous history of speech and language difficulties were reported.

Emily's scores on the PIPA subtests were:

Subtest	Raw score	Standard Score	Percentile
Syllable Segmentation	5/12	8	25
Rhyme Awareness	12/12	15	95
Alliteration Awareness	12/12	14	91
Phoneme Isolation	12/12	12	75
Phoneme Segmentation	8/12	15	95
Letter Knowledge	31/32	14	91

Emily scored above the average range on four of the PIPA subtests. She was within the normal range for phoneme isolation and syllable segmentation. Her syllable segmentation is relatively poor. However the norms indicate that there is a brief stage of development (usually between 5:6 and 6 years of age) when children focus on phonemes at the expense of syllables.

Sean (6 years: 9 months)

Sean had an age equivalent score on the Visual Motor Integration Test (Beery, 1989) of 7 years: 8 months. He lives in rural Yorkshire. No previous history of speech and language difficulties were reported.

Sean's scores on the PIPA subtests were:

Subtest	Raw score	Standard Score	Percentile
Syllable Segmentation	8/12	8	25
Rhyme Awareness	10/12	11	63
Alliteration Awareness	10/12	10	50
Phoneme Isolation	12/12	12	75
Phoneme Segmentation	8/12	14	91
Letter Knowledge	31/32	12	75

Sean scored within the average range on five of the PIPA subtests. He was above average on phoneme segmentation.

Children at risk of literacy problems

Joshua (aged 4 years: 2 months)

Joshua was referred to the Literacy Clinic at the University of Newcastle for an assessment of his speech and literacy skills. He has a history of middle ear infections and has recently had grommets inserted. Joshua had an age equivalent score on the Visual Motor Integration Test (Beery, 1989) of 4 years: 7 months. He has two elder siblings with identified dyslexia.

Joshua presented with delayed speech development. The following speech error patterns were observed: assimilation, weak syllable deletion, stopping, final consonant deletion, cluster reduction and gliding. He has received 10 sessions of individual speech and language therapy.

Joshua's scores on the PIPA subtests were:

Subtest	Raw score	Standard Score	Percentile
Syllable Segmentation	0/12	6	9
Rhyme Awareness	3/12	8	25
Alliteration Awareness	0/12	6	9
Phoneme Isolation	0/12	7	16
Phoneme Segmentation	0/12	8	25
Letter Knowledge	0/32	7	16

Chapter 5

Joshua's performance on the PIPA is at the lower limit of the normal range. However, two indicators that give cause for concern are:

- delayed phonological (speech) development

- limited development of phonological awareness Although at only 4:2 Joshua is as yet not far below what would be expected for his age, his awareness is limited to rhyme. He performed this subtest very slowly, and still scored at chance.

Recommendations: Joshua's spoken phonology and phonological awareness may spontaneously improve. However, he needs to be carefully monitored over a six month period as failure to make progress would indicate a need for intervention.

Liam (aged 5 years: 6 months)

Liam has been assessed at a Speech and Language Therapy Clinic in Brisbane and was on a waiting list for treatment. Liam had an age equivalent score on the Visual Motor Integration Test (Beery, 1989) of 5 years: 6 months.

Liam presented with disordered speech development.

- The following delayed speech error patterns were observed: assimilation, weak syllable deletion, stopping, final consonant deletion and cluster.

- The following deviant error patterns were observed: frication of plosives (e.g., 'ser' for girl), backing of alveolars (e.g., 'karng' for tank) and vowel errors.

Liam's scores on the PIPA subtests were:

Subtest	Raw score	Standard Score	Percentile
Syllable Segmentation	8/12	8	25
Rhyme Awareness	3/12	3	1
Alliteration Awareness	3/12	4	2
Phoneme Isolation	0/12	3	1
Phoneme Segmentation	0/12	7	16

Liam has an uneven performance across the PIPA subtests. Liam presents with some syllabic awareness. His scores on intra-syllabic subtests are poor. Phoneme segmentation skills have yet to develop and need to be monitored.

Recommendations: Liam's spoken phonology should be the focus of therapy and his phonological awareness skills should be carefully monitored. Liam is unlikely to benefit from a general phonological awareness training programme given the deviant nature of his speech error patterns.

James (aged 6 years: 7 months)

James attends a school in a middle SES area of Newcastle. His school was concerned about his lack of progress in reading and spelling. He has no history of speech or language difficulties. His reading ability was assessed with the Schonell Graded reading test (1956). He read nine words accurately which equates to a reading age of 6 years 8 months. His errors on this assessment reveal that James relies on a visual strategy to read single words. For example: sit read as sick, bun read as damp, road read as round. James' ability to use phonic strategies were tested by asking him to complete two subtests from the Queensland University Inventory of Literacy (Dodd, Holm, Oerlemans & McCormick, 1996): non-word reading and spelling. His performance was

Non-word spelling		Non-word reading	
Test item	James' response	Test item	James' response
dorf	foob	acked	kank
lont	lastet	slet	samk
sheve	gotei	bocks	dank
wump	wote	sord	s-o-t-h
suts	satea		

James' scores on the PIPA subtests were:

Subtest	Raw score	Standard Score	Percentile
Syllable Segmentation	10/12	11	63
Rhyme Awareness	3/12	3	1
Alliteration Awareness	1/12	3	1
Phoneme Isolation	8/12	7	16
Phoneme Segmentation	0/12	5	5
Letter Knowledge	10/12	3	1

James' ability to segment words into syllables is age appropriate. His scores on intra-syllabic subtests are relatively poor with the exception of phoneme isolation. This pattern, paired with his reliance on a visual reading strategy and lack of progress would suggest that he is at risk of later literacy problems.

Recommendations: James would be recommended for intervention that targets his intra-syllabic awareness. Following a period of therapy his phonological awareness skills would need to be reviewed using the PIPA so that a comparison to his pre-therapy abilities could be made.

References

Beery, K. (1989). The Developmental Test of Visual Motor Integration. 3rd revision. Cleveland: Modern Curriculum Press.

Bradley, L. & Bryant, P. (1983). Categorizing sounds and learning to read - a causal connection. *Nature, 301*(3), 419–421.

Bryant, P., Bradley, L., MacLean, M. & Crossland, J. (1989). Nursery rhymes, phonological skills and reading. *Journal of Child Language, 16*, 407–428.

Bryant, P. E., MacLean, M., Bradley, L. & Crossland, J. (1990). Rhyme and alliteration, phoneme detection and learning to read. *Developmental Psychology, 26*, 429–438.

Burt, L., Holm, A. & Dodd, B. (1999). Phonological awareness skills of 4-year-old British children: an assessment of developmental data. *International Journal of Language and Communication Disorders, 34*(3), 311–335.

Caravolas, M. & Bruck, M. (1993). The effect of oral and written language input on children's phonological awareness: a cross linguistic study. *Journal of Experimental Child Psychology, 55*, 1–30.

Dodd, B. & Gillon, G. (1997). The nature of the phonological deficit underlying disorders of spoken and written language. In Leong, C. K. Joshi R.M. (eds) *Cross-language Studies of Learning to Read and Spell.* Dordrecht: Kluwer Academic Publishers. pp53–70.

Dodd, B., Holm, A., Oerlemans, M. & McCormick, M. (1996). *Queensland University Inventory of Literacy.* Brisbane: The University of Queensland.

Gathercole, S. & Baddeley, A. (1993). Phonological working memory: a critical building block for reading development and vocabulary acquisition. *European Journal of the Psychology of Education, 8*, 259–272.

Goswami, U. & Bryant, P. (1990). *Phonological Skills and Learning to Read.* Hove: Lawrence Erlbaum Associates.

Hoien, T., Lundberg, I., Stanovich, K. & Bjaalid, I. (1995). Components of phonological awareness. *Reading and Writing, 7*, 171–188.

Johnston, R. & Watson, J. (1997). Developing reading, spelling and phonemic awareness skills in primary school children. *Reading* July, 37–40.

Liberman, I. Y. & Shankweiler, D. (1985). Phonology and the problems of learning to read and write. *Remedial and Special Education, 6*, 8 – 17.

Liberman, I. Y. Shankweiler, D., Fischer, F. W., & Carter, B. (1974). Explicit syllable and phoneme segmentation in the young child. *Journal of Experimental Child Psychology, 18*, 201–212.

Mc Bride-Chang, C. (1995). What is phonological awareness? *Journal of Educational Psychology, 87*, 179– 192.

MacLean, M., Bryant, P. E. & Bradley, L. (1987). Rhymes, nursery rhymes and reading in early childhood. *Merrill-Palmer Quarterly, 33*, 255–282.

References

McCormick, M. (1995). The relationship between the phonological processes in early speech development and later spelling strategies. In B. Dodd (Ed.), *Differential Diagnosis & Treatment of Children with Speech Disorder* (pp. 111–124). London: Whurr Publishers.

Muter, V., Hulme, C. & Snowling, M. (1997) *Phonological Abilities Test*. London: The Psychological Corporation.

Muter, V., Hulme, C., Snowling, M. & Taylor, S. (1998). Segmentation, not rhyming, predicts early progress in learning to read. *Journal of Experimental Child Psychology, 71*, 3–27.

Passenger, T., Stuart, M. & Terrell, C. (2000). Phonological processing and early literacy. *Journal of Reading Research, 23*(1), 55–66.

Rack, J., Snowling, M. & Olsen, R. (1992). The nonword reading deficit in developmental dyslexia: a review. *Reading Research Quarterly, 27*, 28–53.

Read, C. (1971). Pre-school children's knowledge of English phonology. *Harvard Educational Review, 41*, 1–34.

Reid, D. K., Hresko, W. & Hammill, D. (1989). *Test of Early Reading Ability*, Austin Texas: Pro-ed.

Schonell, F, & Schonell, E. (1956). *Diagnostic and attainment testing*. Edinburgh: Oliver & Boyd.

Stuart, M. (1999). Getting reading for reading: Early phoneme awareness and phonics teaching improves reading and spelling in inner-city second language learners. *Journal of Experimental Psychology, 69*, 587–605.

Treiman, R. & Baron, J. (1981). Segmental analysis ability: Development and relation to reading ability. In G. E. MacKinno & T. G. Waller (Eds.). *Reading Research: Advances in Theory and Practice*.159–197 San Diego, California: Academic Press.

Treiman, R. & Zukowski, A. (1996). children's sensitivity to syllables, onsets, rimes and phonemes. *Journal of Experimental Child Psychology, 63*, 193–215.

Yopp, H. K. (1988). The validity and reliability of phonemic awareness tests. *Reading Research Quarterly, 23*(2), 159–177.

Appendices A–D

Appendix A

Subtest standard scores (UK)

3:0 – 3:5 3 years, 0 months, 0 days – 3 years, 5 months, 30 days

Std Score	SSeg	RA	AA	PI	PS	LK	Std Score
17	6–12	7–12	8–12				17
16			7				16
15	5	6	6				15
14	4		5				14
13	3	5	4				13
12		4					12
11	2	3	3				11
10	1	2	2				10
9	0	1	1				9
8			0				8
7		0					7
6							6
5							5
4							4
3							3

Note: It is possible for children in this age group to achieve zero scores and still fall within 1 SD of the mean.

3:6 – 3:11 3 years, 6 months, 0 days – 3 years, 11 months, 30 days

Std Score	SSeg	RA	AA	PI	PS	LK	Std Score
17	9–12	9–12	8–12				17
16	8	8	7				16
15	7	7					15
14	6		6				14
13	5	6	5				13
12		5	4				12
11	4	4					11
10	3	3	3				10
9	2	2	2				9
8	1		1				8
7	0	1					7
6		0	0				6
5							5
4							4
3							3

Note: It is possible for children in this age group to achieve zero scores and still fall within 1 SD of the mean.

Subtest standard scores (UK)

4:0 – 4:5   4 years, 0 months, 0 days – 4 years, 5 months, 30 days

Std Score	SSeg	RA	AA	PI	PS	LK	Std Score
17		12	10–12		6–12	26–33	17
16	12	11	9			24–25	16
15	11	10	8	11–12	5	21–23	15
14	9–10	9	7	10	4	18–20	14
13	8	8		8–9		15–17	13
12	7	7	6	7	3	13–14	12
11	6	6	5	5–6	2	9–12	11
10	5	5	4	4		7–8	10
9	4	4	3	2–3	1	4–6	9
8	3	3	2	1	0	1–3	8
7	2	2	1	0		0	7
6	0–1	1	0				6
5		0					5
4							4
3							3

Note: It is possible for children in this age group to achieve zero scores and still fall within 1 SD of the mean.

4:6 – 4:11   4 years, 6 months, 0 days – 4 years, 11 months, 30 days

Std Score	SSeg	RA	AA	PI	PS	LK	Std Score
17			12		7–12		17
16		12	11				16
15	12	11	10		6	30–32	15
14	10–11	10	9		5	27–29	14
13	9	9	8	11–12	4	23–26	13
12	8	8	7	10		20–22	12
11	7	7	6	8–9	3	16–19	11
10	6	6	5	7	2	13–15	10
9	5	4–5	4	5–6	1	9–12	9
8	3–4	3	3	3–4	0	6–8	8
7	2	2	2	2		2–5	7
6	1	1	0–1	0–1		0–1	6
5	0	0					5
4							4
3							3

Note: SSeg, Syllable Segmentation; RA, Rhyme Awareness; AA, Alliteration Awareness; PI, Phoneme Isolation; PS, Phoneme Segmentation; LK, Letter Knowledge.

Appendix A

Subtest standard scores (UK)

5:0 – 5:5   5 years, 0 months, 0 days – 5 years, 5 months, 30 days

Std Score	SSeg	RA	AA	PI	PS	LK	Std Score
17					10–12		17
16					9		16
15		12			8		15
14	12	11	11–12		7	31–32	14
13	11	10	10		6	28–30	13
12	10	9	9	12	5	25–27	12
11	9	8	8	10–11	4	22–24	11
10	7–8	6–7	6–7	9	3	18–21	10
9	6	5	5	8	2	15–17	9
8	5	4	4	7	1	12–14	8
7	4	3	3	5–6	0	9–11	7
6	3	2	2	4		6–8	6
5	2	1	0–1	3		3–5	5
4	1	0		1–2		0–2	4
3	0			0			3

5:6 – 5:11   5 years, 6 months, 0 days – 5 years, 11 months, 30 days

Std Score	SSeg	RA	AA	PI	PS	LK	Std Score
17							17
16							16
15							15
14		12					14
13		11	12			31–32	13
12	12	10	10–11	12	12	28–30	12
11	10–11	9	9	11	10–11	26–27	11
10	7–9	8	8		7–9	24–25	10
9	5–6	7	7	10	5–6	22–23	9
8	3–4	6	6	9	3–4	19–21	8
7	0–2	5	5	8	0–2	17–18	7
6		4	4			15–16	6
5		3	3	7		12–14	5
4		2	1–2	6		10–11	4
3		0–1	0	0–5		0–9	3

Note: SSeg, Syllable Segmentation; RA, Rhyme Awareness; AA, Alliteration Awareness; PI, Phoneme Isolation; PS, Phoneme Segmentation; LK, Letter Knowledge.

Subtest standard scores (UK)

6:0 – 6:5 6 years, 0 months, 0 days – 6 years, 5 months, 30 days

Std Score	Raw Score SSeg	RA	AA	PI	PS	LK	Std Score
17					10–12		17
16					9		16
15					8		15
14	12	12			7		14
13	11		12			32	13
12	10	11	11	12	6	30–31	12
11	9	10	10	11	5	28–29	11
10	8	9			4	26–27	10
9	7		9	10		25	9
8	6	8	8	9	3	23–24	8
7	5	7	7		2	21–22	7
6	4	6	6	8	1	19–20	6
5	3		5	7		17–18	5
4	2	5	4		0	15–16	4
3	0–1	0–4	0–3	0–6		0–14	3

6:6 – 6:11 6 years, 6 months, 0 days – 6 years, 11 months, 30 days

Std Score	Raw Score SSeg	RA	AA	PI	PS	LK	Std Score
17					10–12		17
16							16
15					9		15
14		12			8		14
13	12		12		7		13
12	11	11		12	6	31–32	12
11	10	10	11	11	5	30	11
10	9	9	10	10		28–29	10
9			9		4	26–27	9
8	8	8	8	9	3	25	8
7	7	7	7	8	2	23–24	7
6	6		6	7	1	22	6
5	5	6	5	6	0	20–21	5
4	4	5				18–19	4
3	0–3	0–4	0–4	0–5		0–17	3

Note: SSeg, Syllable Segmentation; RA, Rhyme Awareness; AA, Alliteration Awareness; PI, Phoneme Isolation; PS, Phoneme Segmentation; LK, Letter Knowledge.

Appendix B

Subtest standard scores (Australia)

3:0 – 3:5 3 years, 0 months, 0 days – 3 years, 5 months, 30 days

Std Score	SSeg	RA	AA	PI	PS	LK	Std Score
17	9–12	7–12	5–12				17
16	8						16
15	7	6					15
14	6		4				14
13	5	5					13
12							12
11	4	4	3				11
10	3	3					10
9	2		2				9
8		2					8
7	1						7
6	0	1	1				6
5							5
4		0					4
3			0				3

3:6 – 3:11 3 years, 6 months, 0 days – 3 years, 11 months, 30 days

Std Score	SSeg	RA	AA	PI	PS	LK	Std Score
17	10–12	10–12	7–12				17
16	9	9					16
15	8	8	6				15
14	7	7					14
13			5				13
12	6	6					12
11	5	5	4				11
10	4	4					10
9	3	3	3				9
8	2	2					8
7		1	2				7
6	1	0	1				6
5	0						5
4			0				4
3							3

Note: SSeg, Syllable Segmentation; RA, Rhyme Awareness; AA, Alliteration Awareness; PI, Phoneme Isolation; PS, Phoneme Segmentation; LK, Letter Knowledge.

Appendix B

Subtest standard scores (Australia)

4:0 – 4:6   4 years, 0 months, 0 days – 4 years, 6 months, 30 days

Std Score	SSeg	RA	AA	PI	PS	LK	Std Score
17	11–12	12	6–12	8–12	3–12		17
16	10	11		7			16
15		10	5	6	2		15
14	9	9		5			14
13	8	8		4			13
12	7	7	4		1		12
11	6	6		3			11
10	5	5	3	2			10
9	4	4		1	0		9
8	3	3	2	0			8
7		2					7
6	2	1					6
5	1	0		1			5
4	0						4
3				0			3

4:6 – 4:11   4 years, 6 months, 0 days – 4 years, 11 months, 30 days

Std Score	SSeg	RA	AA	PI	PS	LK	Std Score
17			11–12		5–12		17
16	12	12	10		4		16
15	11	11	9	11–12			15
14	10	10	8	10	3		14
13	9		7	9			13
12	8	9	6	7–8	2		12
11	7	8	5	6			11
10		7		5	1		10
9	6	6	4	3–4			9
8	5	5	3	2	0		8
7	4	4	2	1			7
6	3	3	1	0			6
5	2	2	0				5
4	1	1					4
3	0	0					3

Note: SSeg, Syllable Segmentation; RA, Rhyme Awareness; AA, Alliteration Awareness; PI, Phoneme Isolation; PS, Phoneme Segmentation; LK, Letter Knowledge.

Appendix B

Subtest standard scores (Australia)

5:0 – 5:5 — 5 years, 0 months, 0 days – 5 years, 5 months, 30 days

Std Score	SSeg	RA	AA	PI	PS	LK	Std Score
17					4–12		17
16			12	12	3		16
15	12		11	11			15
14	11	12	10	10			14
13	10	11	8–9	9	2		13
12	9	10	7	7–8			12
11	8	9	6	6	1		11
10	7	8	5	5			10
9	6	7	4	4			9
8	5	6	3	2–3	0		8
7	4	5	1–2	1			7
6	3	4	0	0			6
5	2	3					5
4	1	2					4
3	0	0–1					3

5:6 – 5:11 — 5 years, 6 months, 0 days – 5 years, 11 months, 30 days

Std Score	SSeg	RA	AA	PI	PS	LK	Std Score
17					10–12		17
16					9		16
15					8		15
14					7		14
13					6		13
12	12		11–12	12	5		12
11	10–11	12	10	11	4		11
10	9	11	9	10	3		10
9	8	9–10	8	9	2		9
8	7	8	7	8	1		8
7	6	7	6	7	0		7
6		6	5	6			6
5	5	5	4	5			5
4	4	4	2–3	4			4
3	0–3	0–3	0–1	0–3			3

Note: SSeg, Syllable Segmentation; RA, Rhyme Awareness; AA, Alliteration Awareness; PI, Phoneme Isolation; PS, Phoneme Segmentation; LK, Letter Knowledge.

Subtest standard scores (Australia)

6:0 – 6:5
6 years, 0 months, 0 days – 6 years, 5 months, 30 days

Std Score	SSeg	RA	AA	PI	PS	LK	Std Score
17					11–12		17
16					10		16
15					9		15
14					8		14
13	12	12			7		13
12	11	11	12	12			12
11	10				6		11
10	9	10			5		10
9	8	9	10–11	11	4		9
8	7	8			3		8
7	6		9		2		7
6		7	8	10	1		6
5	5	6					5
4	4	5	7		0		4
3	0–3	0–4	0–6	0–9			3

6:6 – 6:11
6 years, 6 months, 0 days – 6 years, 11 months, 30 days

Std Score	SSeg	RA	AA	PI	PS	LK	Std Score
17							17
16					12		16
15					11		15
14					10		14
13					9		13
12	12	12	12		8		12
11	11			12	7		11
10	10	11			6		10
9	9				5		9
8	8	10	11	11	4		8
7	7	9			3		7
6				10	2		6
5	6	8			1		5
4	5		10				4
3	0–4	0–7	0–9	0–9	0		3

Note: SSeg, Syllable Segmentation; RA, Rhyme Awareness; AA, Alliteration Awareness; PI, Phoneme Isolation; PS, Phoneme Segmentation; LK, Letter Knowledge.

Appendix C

Confidence intervals +/- standard score points (UK)

Age group	Confidence interval	SSeg	RA	AA	PI	PS	LK	Confidence interval
3:0–3:5	68%	1.5	1.5	0.9				68%
	95%	2.9	2.6	1.7				95%
3:6–3:11	68%	1.0	1.2	1.9				68%
	95%	1.4	2.4	3.8				95%
4:0–4:5	68%	1.1	1.4	1.0	0.4	1.2	0.6	68%
	95%	2.1	2.7	1.9	0.7	2.4	1.2	95%
4:6–4:11	68%	1.2	1.0	1.2	0.4	1.7	0.7	68%
	95%	2.4	1.9	2.4	0.7	3.3	1.3	95%
5:0–5:5	68%	2.1	1.6	2.2	1.5	2.1	0.8	68%
	95%	4.1	3.2	4.4	2.9	4.2	1.6	95%
5:6–5:11	68%	1.7	2.9	1.1	1.5	2.0	0.8	68%
	95%	3.2	5.6	2.1	3.0	3.9	1.5	95%
6:0–6:5	68%	0.9	1.4	1.5	2.1	1.1	1.7	68%
	95%	1.8	2.8	3.0	4.1	2.3	3.3	95%
6:6–6:11	68%	1.4	1.7	1.3	0.3	1.7	0.7	68%
	95%	2.8	3.4	2.6	0.6	3.4	1.4	95%

Note: SSeg, Syllable Segmentation; RA, Rhyme Awareness; AA, Alliteration Awareness; PI, Phoneme Isolation; PS, Phoneme Segmentation; LK, Letter Knowledge.

Percentile ranks corresponding to standard scores

Subtest standard score	Percentile rank
17	99
16	98
15	95
14	91
13	84
12	75
11	63
10	50
9	37
8	25
7	16
6	9
5	5
4	2
3	1